This Notebook Belongs To:

____

83750542R00057

Made in the USA
Columbia, SC
12 December 2017